Urine Dipstick Analysis and Microscopy

Dicken Weatherby, N.D.

Bear Mountain Publishing • Ashland, OR

Urine Dipstick Analysis and Microscopy

Bear Mountain Publishing
1-541-482-3779
ISBN: 0972646914

Warning - Disclaimer

Printed in the United States of America

How to Order

For mail orders call Bear Mountain Publishing in the United States at 541-482-3779, e-mail info@BloodChemistryAnalysis.com or online at http://www.BloodChemistryAnalysis.com

Urine Specific Gravity

Ranges: **Normal Value: 1.015**   **High value: >1.015**   **Low value: <1.015**

Clinical implications   HIGH

Clinical Implication	Additional information
Abnormal solutes in urine	An ⬆ S.G. with ⬆ or normal urine volume. Need to check dipstick to confirm presence of protein or glucose.
Adrenal insufficiency	A high urinary chloride and a high specific gravity is an indication of adrenal insufficiency.
Increased mineral loss	A high specific gravity may be due to increased mineral solutes in the urine.
Diabetes mellitus	Large amounts of glucose or protein ⬆ the S.G. to > 1.050. Note: Every 1% of glucose in the urine will ⬆ the S.G. 0.004
Dehydration	Excess water loss from sweating, fever, vomiting
Other causes of S.G. increase	Hepatic disease, Congestive heart failure, Protein malnutrition, collagen vascular disease

LOW

Clinical Implication	Additional information
Congested lymphatic system	⬇ S.G. and ⬇ or normal urine volume indicates the kidney is having difficulty concentrating the urine and cleansing the blood due to a congested lymphatic system which can cause: swollen glands, allergy symptoms, low back pain, headaches and nausea. Symptoms worsen in women during menses and pregnancy, and may lead to vomiting.
Early chronic renal disease	⬇ S.G. and ⬆ volume
Diabetes insipidus	⬇ S.G. and ⬆⬆ volume
Kidney inflammation and infection	⬇ S.G. and ⬇ volume Glomerulonephritis (inflammation without infection) Pyelonephritis (inflammation with infection)

Urine Bilirubin

Normal values: Zero

Clinical implications
Even trace amounts of urinary bilirubin are abnormal and therefore further testing is indicated.
Positive reading

Clinical Implication	Additional information	
Gall bladder dysfunction	Biliary stasis or gallstones. Further testing should be performed to assess this situation.	
Protein maldigestion	This can interfere with the transport of bilirubin into the small intestine.	
Oxidative stress	Excess red blood cell destruction, leading to increased bilirubin levels, may be caused by increased oxidative stress	
Liver detox stress	Consider phase II liver detoxification problems	
Liver dysfunction (Inflammation or infection causing conjugation problems)	• Infectious hepatitis • Cirrhosis of the liver • Metastatic disease of the liver • Congestive heart failure	• Gilbert's disease • Jaundice • Other liver diseases caused by toxic or infectious agents

Note: Urine bilirubin is negative in hemolytic diseases

More comprehensive diagnostic information can be obtained by comparing urine bilirubin with urine urobilinogen levels:

Bilirubin	Urobilinogen	Clinical Implication
↑	↑	Liver dysfunction, hepatocellular or partial obstruction
↑	Normal	Biliary stasis or gall stones
Negative	↑	Hemolytic
Negative	Normal	Negative

Urine Blood or Hemoglobin

Normal levels: None

Clinical implications
Hematuria
Non-Hemolyzed

Clinical Implication	Additional information
Conditions associated with hematuria	<ul><li>Lower urinary tract infections</li><li>Kidney stones</li><li>Hypertension</li><li>Allergies</li><li>Urinary tract or kidney cancer</li><li>Glomerular infection or inflammation</li><li>Lupus</li><li>Heavy smokers</li><li>Trauma</li></ul>

Hemolyzed

Clinical Implication	Additional information
Oxidative stress	Oxidation and breakdown of red blood cells causes an increase in hemolysed blood. Check Oxidata test.
Other conditions	<ul><li>Liver pathology</li><li>Allergies</li></ul>

Urine Color

Normal values: The color of the urine is straw to amber

Color of Urine	Clinical Implications	
Colorless	• Large fluid intake • Diabetes insipidus • Untreated diabetes mellitus	• Alcohol ingestion • Severe iron deficiency • Chronic interstitial nephritis
Orange-colored	• Concentrated urine (inadequate fluid intake, excessive fluid loss, fever) • Bile • Drugs (pyridium, rifampin, aco-gantrisin, furoxone, dilantin)	• Diet (carrot juice, carotenes, riboflavin, food dyes) • Uric acid crystals
Brownish color or greenish yellow	• Bilirubin in urine • Biliverdin (oxidation of bilirubin on standing), drugs (methylene blue, elavil), indican, pseudomonas infection	
Red (straw to port wine)	• Blood, hemoglobin, or myoglobin, • Porphyria (port wine color), • Drugs: phenophthaleins, dorbane (laxative),	• Diet (beets, blackberries), • Herbs: cascara, senna, • Aniline dyes
Brown	• Blood (acid hematin), • Bilirubin and other bile pigments (yellow-brown to yellow green). • Urobilinogen, • Melanin (melanogin conversion by exposure to light in multiple myeloma, melanotic tumor, addison's disease),	• Indican, • Phenols, • Drugs (flagyl, nitrofurantoin, l-dopa, methyldopa, metronidazole, sulfonamides), lysol poisoning (brown-black), • Rhubarb
Blue hue	• Food dyes • Medication	• Pseudomonas infection • Some porphyries
Green	• Pseudomonas infection	

Urine Glucose

Normal value: Negative

Clinical implications   HIGH

Clinical Implication	Additional information	
Glycosuria with high blood sugars	1. Diabetes mellitus (also ↑ S.G.) 2. Endocrine diseases 3. Infections	4. Extreme emotional stress 5. Obesity 6. Diabetes insipidus
Glycosuria without a high blood sugar	1. Renal tubule disease (lowered renal threshold) 2. Pregnancy 3. Heavy metal poisoning	4. Fanconi's syndrome (amino acid reabsorption defect) 5. Inflammatory renal disease

Urine Ketones

Normal value: Negative

Clinical implications   HIGH (Ketosis)

Clinical Implication	Additional information	
Low carbohydrate, & high fat/protein diets	Ketones often get produced in these types of diets due to the lack of carbohydrate consumed (Zone and Atkins type diets)	
Liver dysfunction	Ketosis often occurs with a decreased liver glycogen. There may also be adrenal hypofunction, as cortisol is needed to stimulate the liver to release glycogen.	
Dietary conditions	1. Increased fat intake or inability to metabolize fats 2. Starvation and fasting 3. Prolonged vomiting	4. Anorexia 5. Increased protein intake
Carbohydrate maldigestion	This is especially true if the patient is eating carbohydrates and there are ketones in the urine	
Kidney disease or kidney failure	Renal glycosuria	
Blood sugar abnormalities	1. Diabetic acidosis	2. Severe hypoglycemia
Dehydration	Kidneys are unable to eliminate ketones efficiently	
Increased metabolic states	1. Hyperthyroidism 2. Fever	2. Pregnancy or lactation

Urine Leukocyte Esterase

Normal values: Zero. A color change occurs with > 5 WBCs/high powered field

Clinical implications	Positive reading	
Clinical Implication	**Additional information**	
Infection or inflammation	• Intestinal inflammation • Pyelonephritis (acute or chronic) • Cystitis or Urethritis	• Prostatitis • Kidney stones • Acute glomerulonephritis
Other causes for the presence of leukocyte esterase	• retained foreign body • Dehydration	• Fever • Stress

Urine Nitrites

Normal value: Negative for bacteria

Clinical implications	Positive reading
Clinical Implication	**Additional information**
Bacteriauria	A positive nitrite test indicates the presence of bacteria in the urine, suggesting a urinary tract infection. This test does not confirm an infection, so further testing in the form of microscopic evaluation of urine and urine culture needs to be performed.

↑ Nitrites along with an ↑ Leukocyte esterase = infection

Urine Odor

Normal values: Urine is normally odorless

Ammonia/fetid	• Presence of bacterial overgrowth	• Loss of alkaline buffers in the body
Sweetish, brown, frothy	• Presence of bile (bile duct obstruction)	
Sweet	• Look for sugar problems e.g. diabetes	• Biliary problems
Fruity and sweet	• Ketoneuria	
Foul	• Fecal contamination, recto-urethral fistula	
Mousy, musty	• Phenylketonuria	
Maple syrup	• Maple syrup urine disease	
Any strong, unusual, persistent odor	• Maybe herbs or medications • Metabolic disorders	

Urine Protein

Normal Ranges: Negative or trace

Proteinuria

Glomerular damage	Proteinuria is usually the result of an increased glomerular filtration rate	
Renal diseases	• Nephritis/glomerulonephritis, • Nephrosis, • Malignant hypertension,	• Polycystic kidneys, • Chronic urinary tract obstruction
Non-renal diseases	• Allergies • Fever, • Acute infection, • Leukemia/multiple myeloma	• Toxemia • Diabetes mellitus • SLE
↑ **Protein and** ↑ **Leukocytes**	Usually an infection at some level in the urinary tract	

Urine Turbidity or Appearance

Normal values: Fresh urine is clear to slightly hazy

Hazy	1. Cooling of the sample, 2. Ph change,	3. RBC's
Cloudy urine- unable to see through the sample	1. Amorphous sediment or amorphous crystals , depending on urine ph (phosphates with alkaline urine, urates with acidic urine) 2. Pus, with WBC count > 200 cells / mm3 3. Blood, with RBC count > 500 cells / mm3 4. Epithelial cells 5. Bacteria 6. Fat - milky appearance	7. Chylomicrons - creamy color - obstruction of lymph vessels by parasites, thoracic duct obstruction, trauma, or tumor 8. Conjugated bilirubin - parenchymal liver disease, biliary tract obstruction 9. Urobilinogen - parenchymal liver disease, hemolytic disease 10. Oxalic or glycolic acids 11. Mucus

Urine Urobilinogen

Normal Ranges: Trace

HIGH

Clinical Implication	Additional information	
Increased destruction of blood cells	• Hemolytic anemia • Pernicious anemia • Malaria	• ↑ Xenotoxins • Infections • ↑ Oxidative stress
Hemorrhage into the tissues	• Pulmonary infarct	• Excessive bruising
Reduced conjugation of bilirubin by the liver **↑ Toxins in the body**	↑ Urobilinogen is a sign that the liver is not functioning very well	
Hepatic damage as a result of:	• Gall bladder disease- biliary obstruction • Cirrhosis	• Acute hepatitis
Check all conditions that affect blood break down		

LOW

Clinical Implication	Additional information	
Anything that prevents bilirubin excretion into the intestines	• Gall stones • Biliary stasis	• Severe inflammation of biliary ducts • Cancer of the head of the pancreas
Antibiotic therapy	Antibiotics wipe out the normal digestive flora which may prevent the formation of urobilinogen from bilirubin	

Interfering Factors: **Diurnal variation:** Peak excretion occurs from noon to 4:00 PM
More comprehensive diagnostic information can be obtained by comparing urine urobilinogen with urine bilirubin levels:

Bilirubin	Urobilinogen	Clinical Implication
↑	↑	Liver dysfunction, hepatocellular or partial obstruction
↑	Normal	Biliary stasis or gall stones
Negative	↑	Hemolytic
Negative	Normal	Negative

Urine Volume

Ranges for a 24-hour sample:

Normal volume: 800-2000ml	Polyuria: > 2400ml	Oliguria: <800ml
Abnormal solutes: >1800ml with S.G.>1.020	Poor kidney conc.: <1400ml with S.G.<1.020	The average value: 1500 ml.

HIGH (>2400ml)

Clinical Implication	Additional information	
Eating a junk food diet	Junk food diets or Standard American Diets can have a diuretic effect on then body causing a mild polyuria	
Ingested diuretics	Taking of diuretic medications and the consumption of tea, coffee, soda, alcohol etc. can cause polyuria	
Other functional problems	1. Allergies	2. Underactive adrenals
Polyuria- with ↑ BUN and creatinine levels	1. Diabetic ketoacidosis,	2. Partial obstruction of urinary tract
Polyuria with normal BUN and creatinine levels	1. Diabetes mellitus 2. Diabetes insipidus	3. Certain tumors of brain and spinal cord

LOW (<800ml)

Clinical Implication	Additional information	
Renal causes	1. Renal ischemia 2. Glomerulonephritis and nephritis	3. Renal disease caused by toxic agent
Dehydration	Cause by prolonged vomiting, diarrhea or excess sweating	
Other causes of oliguria	Over active adrenals, edema, recovering from fever, urinary tract obstruction, cardiac insufficiency	

Urinary Microscopy

Discussion

Urine microscopy is performed on the sediment of urine that has been centrifuged. The sediment is evaluated for cellular elements (red and white blood cells and epithelial cells), casts, crystals and bacteria which might originate from anywhere in the genitourinary tract.

When would you run this test?

1. To investigate and further evaluate positive findings from the Urine reagent dipstick testing

	Discussion	Normal	Clinical implications	Interfering factors
RBCs	RBCs occasionally can be found in the urine. Persistent findings of even small amounts of erythrocytes should be investigated because they come from the kidney and may signal serious renal dysfunction. They are usually diagnostic for glomerular diseases.	0-2/HPF normal >2 is abnormal and needs to be investigated	• Renal or systemic disease • Trauma to kidneys • Kidney stones • Pyelonephritis • Cystitis • Prostatitis	Alkaline urine hemolyzes red blood cells Heavy smokers have small amounts of RBCs in urine Menstruation Strenuous exercise
Red cell casts	Red cell casts indicate acute inflammatory or vascular disorders in the glomerulus. Their presence in the urine may be the only manifestation of certain diseases.	Zero casts	• Acute glomerulonephritis (GN) • Associated with SLE	May appear after strenuous physical activity or contact sports Alkaline urine dissolves RBC casts
WBCs	WBCs may originate from anywhere in the genitourinary tract	0-4/HPF	• >50/HPF indicates acute bacterial infection within urinary tract (perform urine culture) • All renal diseases • Cystitis or prostatitis • Chronic pyelonephritis (PN)	Strenuous exercise Vaginal discharge- need clean catch
WBC casts	Always come from the kidney tubules Indicates renal parenchymal infection	Zero casts	• PN (most common cause) • Occasionally acute GN	
Epithelial cells	Cells from the kidneys, bladder or urethra and vagina (squamous)	0-2/HPF (renal) Squamous are common	• Acute tubular damage • Acute GN	

	Discussion	Normal	Clinical implications	Interfering factors
Epithelial cell casts	Caused by the cast-off tubule cells in the kidney that slowly degenerates. Will appear in large numbers when there is damage to tubule epithelium	Zero	• Nephrosis • GN	
Bacteria	Increased amounts are seen with renal and urinary tract infections	Small amounts in non-clean catch	20 or more bacteria per high powered microscope field may indicate a UTI (do urine culture)	Non-clean catch
Yeast	Usually indicates vaginal contamination	Zero	In males: immunosupression	Non-clean catch
Hyaline casts	Formed from precipitation of protein within the tubules. Their presence depends on flow of urine, urine pH and if present degree of proteinuria. Usually non pathological	0-2/LPF	non-pathological, form after exercise or in concentrated or highly acidic urine With proteinuria Indicates possible damage to glomerular membrane, which permits leakage of proteins: Nephritis Malignant HTN Chronic renal disease	

Urine Crystals

May present with no symptoms or are associated with kidney stone formation. The type of crystal formed varies with urine pH.

Type of Crystal	Ph of urine	Clinical implication
Uric acid	5.0-6.5	gout, acute febrile conditions, chronic nephritis
Amorphous urates, sodium urate	5.0-6.5	salts of Na+, K+, Mg++, Ca++; normal
Calcium oxalate	Up to pH 7.5	Fat digestion problems, ethylene glycol poisoning, DM, liver disease, severe renal disease, ingestion of oxalate-rich foods
Cystine	5.0-6.5	pathological ; indicates an inherited metabolic condition
Leucine	5.0-6.5	pathological ; maple syrup or oathouse urine disease, liver disease
Tyrosine	5.0-6.5	pathological ; tyrosinosis, Oathouse urine disease, liver disease
Hippuric acid	5.0-6.5	no significance
Cholesterol	5.0-6.5	indicates excessive tissue breakdown - nephrotic syndrome, chyluria (fat in urine), filariasis, tumors
Triple phosphates	7.5-9.0	ammonium-magnesium-phosphate - with urinary calculi, chronic pyelitis, chronic cystitis, BPH with urinary retention
Amorphous phosphates	7.5-9.0	similar to amorphous urates ; no significance
Calcium carbonate	7.5-9.0	no significance
Calcium phosphate	7.5-9.0	may form calculi
Ammonium urate	7.5-9.0	found with bacterial infection if in freshly voided urine

Urine Dipstick Results form

Client's Name: _____   Practitioner: _____

Pathology Screening With Reagent Test Strip   Date: _____

TEST	NORMAL	ABNORMAL FINDINGS				
Color	Straw to amber	Colorless	red	green/yellow	orange	brown
Turbidity	Clear to hazy	Cloudy	very cloudy		mucous	
Volume	1500 ml	< 800ml (oliguria)			> 2400ml (polyuria)	
Glucose	Negative	+1	+2	+3	+4	
Bilirubin	Negative	+1	+2	+3		
Ketones	Negative	+1	+2	+3		
Blood	Negative	**Hemolyzed:** +1 (5-10)	+2 (10-25)	+3 (25-50)	+4 (>50)	
		Non-heme.: +1 (5-10)	+2 (10-25)	+3 (25-50)	+4 (>50)	
Protein	Negative	Trace (5-20mg) +1 (30mg)	+2 (100mg)	+3 (300mg) +4		
Urobilinogen	Trace	+1	+2	+3	+4	
Nitrites	Negative	Positive				
Leukocytes	Negative	+1 (10-25)	+2 (25-75)	+3 (>75)		

Pathology Screening With Reagent Test Strip   Date: _____

TEST	NORMAL	ABNORMAL FINDINGS				
Color	Straw to amber	Colorless	red	green/yellow	orange	brown
Turbidity	Clear to hazy	Cloudy	very cloudy		mucous	
Volume	1500 ml	< 800ml (oliguria)			> 2400ml (polyuria)	
Glucose	Negative	+1	+2	+3	+4	
Bilirubin	Negative	+1	+2	+3		
Ketones	Negative	+1	+2	+3		
Blood	Negative	**Hemolyzed:** +1 (5-10)	+2 (10-25)	+3 (25-50)	+4 (>50)	
		Non-heme.: +1 (5-10)	+2 (10-25)	+3 (25-50)	+4 (>50)	
Protein	Negative	Trace (5-20mg) +1 (30mg)	+2 (100mg)	+3 (300mg) +4		
Urobilinogen	Trace	+1	+2	+3	+4	
Nitrites	Negative	Positive				
Leukocytes	Negative	+1 (10-25)	+2 (25-75)	+3 (>75)		

Pathology Screening With Reagent Test Strip   Date: _____

TEST	NORMAL	ABNORMAL FINDINGS				
Color	Straw to amber	Colorless	red	green/yellow	orange	brown
Turbidity	Clear to hazy	Cloudy	very cloudy		mucous	
Volume	1500 ml	< 800ml (oliguria)			> 2400ml (polyuria)	
Glucose	Negative	+1	+2	+3	+4	
Bilirubin	Negative	+1	+2	+3		
Ketones	Negative	+1	+2	+3		
Blood	Negative	**Hemolyzed:** +1 (5-10)	+2 (10-25)	+3 (25-50)	+4 (>50)	
		Non-heme.: +1 (5-10)	+2 (10-25)	+3 (25-50)	+4 (>50)	
Protein	Negative	Trace (5-20mg) +1 (30mg)	+2 (100mg)	+3 (300mg) +4		
Urobilinogen	Trace	+1	+2	+3	+4	
Nitrites	Negative	Positive				
Leukocytes	Negative	+1 (10-25)	+2 (25-75)	+3 (>75)		

www.BloodChemistryAnalysis.com

Quick Reference Guide to Functional Urinalysis

And Other In-Office Tests

Dicken Weatherby, N.D.

Bear Mountain Publishing • Ashland, OR

Quick Reference Guide to Functional Urinalysis

Bear Mountain Publishing
1-541-482-3779

Warning - Disclaimer

Bear Mountain Publishing has designed this book to provide information in regard to the subject matter covered. It is sold with the understanding that the publisher and the authors are not liable for the misconception or misuse of information provided. The purpose of this book is to educate. It is not meant to be a comprehensive source for diagnostic testing, and is not intended as a substitute for medical diagnosis or treatment, or intended as a substitute for medical counseling. Information contained in this book should not be construed as a claim or representation that any treatment, process or interpretation mentioned constitutes a cure, palliative, or ameliorative. The interpretation is intended to supplement the practitioner's knowledge of their patient. It should be considered as adjunctive support to other diagnostic medical procedures.

Printed in the United States of America

How to Order

For mail orders call Bear Mountain Publishing in the United States at 541-482-3779, e-mail info@BloodChemistryAnalysis.com or online at http://www.BloodChemistryAnalysis.com

Introduction

This section focuses on the patterns or combinations that exist between 2 or more elements and the diagnostic information that can be found with such an analysis.

When analyzing the patterns it might be useful to look back at each of the individual component.

The following is a glossary of terms that are used in describing some of these patterns:

Digestion: The breakdown of food particles in the GI tract

Absorption: Passage of food particles across the intestinal mucosa

Assimilation: Nutrients are assimilated into the blood stream

Utilization: Passage of nutrients from the blood through the cell membrane

1. **Assimilation and digestion**
2. **Acid/Alkaline Assessment**
3. **Electrolyte assessment**
4. **Calcium and mineralization**
5. **Macronutrient Maldigestion Patterns**
6. **Urine bilirubin with urine urobilinogen levels**

Assimilation and digestion

PATTERN	INTERPRETATION	CLINICAL IMPLICATIONS
↑ Indican ↑ Sediment	Hypochlorhydria Pancreatic Insufficiency Leaky Gut Syndrome	1. High indican levels are a reflection of protein mal-digestion and an excess of undigested food particles. Both of these are signs of hypochlorhydria. 2. High sediment reflects poor breakdown of the absorbed nutrients due to leaky gut syndrome or pancreatic insufficiency (lack or decreased activity of digestive enzymes). Patients with this pattern may inform you that their appetite is extremely high and that they eat even when they are not hungry.
↑ Indican ↕ Sediment	Maldigestion Malabsorption	This pattern indicates poor digestion and absorption of nutrients across the gut wall into the blood and cell. There may be damage to the small intestine mucosa, as a result of a bacterial overgrowth or other infection, causing decreased permeability or a reduced intestinal mucosal surface area. One of the symptoms of this might be an excessive appetite. The maldigestion may be from hypochlorhydria or pancreatic insufficiency.
N indican ↓ Sediment	Malabsorption Deficient Dietary intake	This pattern indicates malabsorption without maldigestion. There may also be a relatively deficient dietary intake as a result of poor diet or a relative reduction in food intake. There may be damage to the small intestine mucosa.
N indican ↑ Sediment	Leaky Gut Syndrome Vitamin/mineral deficiencies	This pattern indicates good digestion but an increased permeability. With increased sediment there is evidence of abnormal metabolites being absorbed through a leaky gut. The increase in abnormal metabolites may be due to a deficiency in minerals and vitamins that act as co-enzymes to the enzymatic processes of digestion. This is a pattern often seen in people who are eating large amounts of one food group
↑ Indican ↑ Calcium	Hypochlorhydria	This pattern is associated with poor digestion, especially proteins, due to an inability to produce enough acidity in the stomach i.e. Hypochlorhydria. Since half of the circulating calcium is bound to protein, a protein deficiency resulting from an HCL deficiency could increase the ionized (diffusible) calcium, which is readily excreted in the urine.
↑ Indican ↓ Calcium	Lowered systemic pH Bicarbonate deficiency ↑ Phosphorous loss	This pattern may suggest a high loss of phosphorous due to increased systemic acidity. This may be result from a deficiency in bicarbonate buffers. There is decreased calcium because it is being used to buffer excess hydrogen ions in the extracellular fluid.

Acid/Alkaline Assessment

PATTERN	INTERPRETATION	CLINICAL IMPLICATIONS
↑ Resp. rate ↓ Breath hold ↓ Urine pH ↑ Saliva pH	Metabolic Acidosis	1. Alkaline saliva- the respiratory system kicks in by increasing the rate and depth of breathing to blow off as much CO2 as possible. This will lower the carbonic acid levels in the body leading to alkaline saliva. 2. Acidic urine- this represents the kidney excreting H+ 3. Increased respiratory rate- The body is attempting to blow off CO2 to decrease carbonic acid levels 4. Decreased breath holding time- acidosis causes a decreased oxygen transport and uptake, thus leading to a decreased ability to hold ones breath
↑/↓ Resp. rate ↓ Breath hold ↓ Urine pH ↓ Saliva pH	Respiratory Acidosis	1. Acid saliva- due to the increased levels of CO2 and carbonic acid 2. Acidic urine- due to the kidney excretion of H+ 3. Increased respiratory rate- The body is attempting to blow off CO2 to decrease carbonic acid levels that have built up as a result of the hypoventilation, which is a hallmark of respiratory acidosis 4. Decreased breath holding time- acidosis causes a decreased oxygen transport and uptake, thus leading to a decreased ability to hold ones breath
↑/↓ Resp. rate ↑ Breath hold ↑ Urine pH ↑ Saliva pH	Respiratory Alkalosis (Also known as stress or anxiety alkalosis)	1. Alkaline saliva- due to the increased loss of CO2 and carbonic acid 2. Alkaline urine- due to the kidney retention of H+ 3. The respiratory rate may be increased or decreased- The body is attempting to blow off CO2 to decrease carbonic acid levels but the respiration patterns are often irregular 4. Increased breath holding time- alkalosis causes an increased oxygen transport and uptake, thus leading to an increased ability to hold ones breath
↓ Resp. rate ↑ Breath hold ↑ Urine pH ↓ Saliva pH	Metabolic alkalosis	1. Acidic saliva- a slowing of the respiration rate will cause more carbonic acid in the extracellular fluids leading to an acidic saliva 2. Alkaline urine- due to kidney excretion of bicarbonate and retention H+ 3. Decreased respiratory rate- due to the suppression of the respiratory centers (the body is attempting to lessen the blow off CO2 to increase carbonic acid levels) 4. Increased breath holding time- alkalosis causes an increased oxygen transport and uptake, thus leading to an increased ability to hold ones breath

Electrolyte assessment

PATTERN	INTERPRETATION	CLINICAL IMPLICATIONS
↓ Urine chloride ↑ Urine pH	Excess alkaline reserves	The extracellular fluid is alkaline. Large amounts of chloride are reabsorbed resulting in a decreased urine chloride. The renal tubules release bicarbonate and hold onto H+ in order to buffer the excess alkalinity. The urine becomes alkaline. This is a normal variation.
↑ Urine chloride ↓ Urine pH	Excess acid reserves Electrolyte insufficiency	The extracellular fluid is acidic. The body copes by causing the renal tubules to reabsorb bicarbonate in order to buffer the acidity. Urine becomes more acidic. Chloride ion reabsorption is decreased resulting in a high urine chloride. This is a normal variation.
↓ Urine chloride ↓ Urine pH	Potassium deficiency Salt deficiency	The blood is deficient in potassium, from eating the standard American diet, too much refined sugar or diuretic use, produces this pattern. The body is excreting H+ and retaining chloride, which leads to an acidic urine. Because of the low pH the body excretes more potassium. If patient has this pattern and reports that their urine output is low consider sodium deficiency because the body is retaining chloride and excreting H+.
↑ Urine chloride ↑ Urine pH ↑ Calcium	Excess salt	In this pattern the body is excreting bicarbonate and chloride as well as calcium. This pattern is seen in people who consume excess amounts of salt.
↑ Urine chloride ↑ Urine pH ↓ Calcium	Excess potassium	This pattern is similar but different from the one above. In this pattern the body is excreting bicarbonate and chloride, but retaining calcium. This pattern is seen in salt deficient diets or people who are taking too much potassium.

Calcium and mineralization

PATTERN	INTERPRETATION	CLINICAL IMPLICATIONS
↓ Urine pH ↓ Calcium	**Excess stomach acid**	Excess stomach acid- possible causes often associated with this pattern are: • Very high protein diet • Magnesium deficiency, because magnesium neutralizes HCl in the stomach. • Medications • Taking Betaine HCl • Acid retention due to kidney disease • Ketosis from fasting or diabetes
↓Urine pH ↑ Calcium	**Complex carbohydrate deficiency** **Alkaline mineral deficiency**	Complex carbohydrate deficiency associated with the standard American Diet i.e. fast food diet high in sugar and protein (↑ sugar can cause ↑ calcium in the urine) Alkaline minerals are being depleted in order to alkalinize the cell. A pattern seen in respiratory acidosis and respiratory conditions such as asthma and emphysema. You may see this pattern after an acute asthma attack.
↑ Urine pH ↓ Calcium	**Hypochlorhydria**	Hypochlorhydria can cause poor protein digestion leading to low calcium levels since half of the calcium is bound to protein. It is also suggestive of the following: • Poor protein and calcium digestion and transportation due to Hypochlorhydria • Poor reserve levels of calcium in the bones • Fatty acid deficiency.
↑ Urine pH ↑ Calcium	**Protein deficiency**	This pattern can be due to protein deficiency due to low protein diet or poor protein absorption. Use of protease to increase absorption may be useful. The increase in calcium may be due to the intake of a non-ionizing form of calcium
N Urine pH ↓ Calcium	**Low calcium levels in body**	May be caused by insufficient intake of calcium or other factors that affect calcium digestion, absorption and utilization. Most of the unabsorbed calcium will be excreted in the stool.

Macronutrient Maldigestion Patterns

PATTERN	INTERPRETATION	CLINICAL IMPLICATIONS
↓ Urine chloride ↑ S.G.	Protein maldigestion	This pattern indicates a difficulty in digesting protein either from a deficiency in protease enzyme or hypochlorhydria. This is associated with a loss of muscle mass, poor recovery time after exercise, hypoglycemia/blood sugar dysregulation, and poor utilization of calcium and magnesium, which must bind with amino acids to be fully assimilated. People with this pattern may also have intestinal mucosal integrity problems causing ileocecal valve problems, constipation and other lower bowel problems. This may be due to glutamine deficiencies.
↓ Urine chloride ↓ S.G.	Fat maldigestion	This pattern indicates a difficulty in dealing with fats either from a deficiency in lipase enzymes or poor bile emulsification. Your patients may talk about having a fat intolerance. This is associated with a deficiency in essential fatty acids, fat soluble nutrient deficiencies and liver and/or gallbladder problems.
↑ Urine chloride ↑ S.G.	Fiber and carbohydrate maldigestion	This pattern indicates fiber and carbohydrate maldigestion and metabolism, which may result from a deficiency in amylase or cellulase, or a high carbohydrate, low protein, low sodium and low fat diet. This pattern is associated with irritable bowel like symptoms, such as diarrhea. With this combination the pituitary increases the stimulation of ADH and GH to retain electrolytes. The patient may suffer from poor circulation, cold hands and feet, and a low sex drive.
↑ Urine chloride ↓ S.G.	Sugar maldigestion	This pattern is common in people who have problem digesting and handling sugar. Patients may consume large amounts of carbohydrates and say that they are sugar intolerant. This pattern is associated with the following conditions: • Sugar handling difficulties • Malabsorption, • Decreased cell permeability Sugar intolerance may also lead to depression, insomnia, emotional instability, and panic attacks.

Urine bilirubin with urine urobilinogen levels

PATTERN	INTERPRETATION	CLINICAL IMPLICATIONS
↑ bilirubin ↑ Urobilinogen	Liver dysfunction	This pattern has its origin in the liver with possible hepatocellular dysfunction or partial obstruction
↑ Bilirubin N Urobilinogen	Biliary Stasis	This pattern is associated with more of a gallbladder origin either biliary stasis with congested bile or gall stones
Neg Bilirubin ↑ Urobilinogen	Hemolytic in origin	This pattern is more hemolytic in origin. There is an increase in red blood cell destruction due to hemolytic anemia, oxidative stress, ↑ xenotoxins.

Other patterns:

Increased Oxidative Stress	↑ Oxidata test ↑ Urinary urobilinogen ↑ Hemolysed blood in urine

CONDITIONS AND TERRAIN ASSESSMENT TESTS

CONDITION	HIGH	LOW
Adrenal hyperfunctioning		↓ Urine chloride
Adrenal hypofunctioning	↑ Urine chloride	
Alkaline mineral insufficiency	↑ Saliva pH ↑ Calcium oxalate sediment ↑ Urine chloride	↓ Saliva pH
Antioxidant insufficiency	↑ Oxidata test	
Bowel toxemia	↑ Indican	
Carbohydrate maldigestion	↑ Calcium phos. sediment ↑ Urine chloride ↑ Specific gravity ↑ Urine ketones	↓ Urine pH ↓ Saliva pH
Complex carbohydrate deficiency	↑ Urine Calcium	↓ Urine pH
Deficient dietary intake	Normal Indican	↓ Total sediment
Dysbiosis	↑ Indican	
Electrolyte insufficiency	↑ Urine chloride	↓ Urine pH
Electrolyte stress	↑ Urine pH	↓ Urine chloride
Essential fatty acid deficiency		↓ Saliva pH
Excess protein intake	↑ Indican ↑ Uric acid sediment ↑ Urine ketones	↓ Urine calcium ↓ Urine pH

CONDITION	HIGH	LOW
Fat maldigestion	↑ Indican ↑ Calcium oxalate sediment	↓ Urine pH ↓ Saliva pH ↓ Urine chloride ↓ Specific gravity
Gallbladder insufficiency	↑ Calcium oxalate sediment ↑ Urine Bilirubin	
Hypochlorhydria	↑ Saliva pH ↑ Indican ↑ Uric acid sediment ↑ Urine chloride ↑ Urine pH	↓ Urine calcium
Hypothyroidism, Subclinical		↓ Basal body temp ↓ Iodine ↓ Achilles return reflex
Immune dysfunction	↑ Urine pH	
Iodine insufficiency		↓ Iodine
Kidney stress	↑ 1st AM Urine pH ↑ Urine chloride ↑ Oxidata test	
Leaky gut syndrome	↑ Total sediment ↑ Indican	
Liver stress	↑ 1st AM Urine pH ↑ Urine bilirubin ↑ Urine ketones ↑ Urine urobilinogen	
Low calcium levels		↓ Urine calcium
Low redox potential		↓ Oxidata test
Malabsorption	↑ Indican	↓ Saliva pH ↓ Total urine sediment ↓ Urine chloride

CONDITION	HIGH	LOW
Maldigestion	↑ Saliva pH ↑ Indican ↑ Oxidata test	↓ Urine pH ↓ Total sediment
Metabolic acidosis	↑ Respiration rate ↑ Saliva pH	↓ Breath holding time ↓ Urine pH ↓ Calcium
Metabolic alkalosis	↑ Breath holding time ↑ Urine pH ↑ Calcium	↓ Respiration rate ↓ Saliva pH
Oxidative stress	↑ Oxidata test ↑ Urine chloride ↑ Urine bilirubin ↑ Urine urobilinogen ↑ Urine blood- hemolysed	
Pancreatic insufficiency	↑ Total sediment	↓ Urine pH ↓ Saliva pH
Protein deficiency	↑ Urine pH ↑ Urine calcium	
Protein maldigestion	↑ Urine pH ↑ Indican ↑ Uric acid sediment ↑ Specific gravity ↑ Urine bilirubin	↓ Urine chloride
Respiratory acidosis	↑ Respiration rate ↑ Urine calcium	↓ Respiration rate ↓ Breath holding time ↓ Urine pH ↓ Saliva pH
Respiratory alkalosis	↑ Respiration rate ↑ Breath holding time ↑ Saliva pH ↑ Urine pH	↓ Respiration rate ↓ calcium

INDIVIDUAL TESTS

Acid-base Terrain

Tests used to identify patterns of acid/alkaline imbalance

↑ Breath hold	↑ Resp. Rate	↑ Urine pH	↑ Saliva pH
• Metabolic alkalosis • Respiratory alkalosis	• Metabolic acidosis • Respiratory acidosis (compensation) • Respiratory alkalosis (acute) • Sympathetic stress	• Bacterial infection • Susceptibility to yeast and viruses • Protein maldigestion • Alkalosis (respiratory and metabolic) • Calcium metabolism problems	• Metabolic acidosis • Respiratory alkalosis • Maldigestion • Hypochlorhydria • Sympathetic dominance • Alkaline mineral insufficiency • Dental tartar

↓ Breath hold	↓ Resp. Rate	↓ Urine pH	↓ Saliva pH
• Metabolic acidosis • Respiratory acidosis • Anemia • Antioxidant insufficiency • Anxiety • Stress	• Metabolic alkalosis • Respiratory acidosis (acute/primary cause) • Respiratory alkalosis (Compensation)	• Maldigestion • Carbohydrate and fat maldigestion • Phase III detoxification issues • Pancreatic insufficiency • Acidosis (respiratory and metabolic) • Inflammation • Arthritis	• Metabolic alkalosis • Respiratory acidosis • Malabsorption • Carbohydrate maldigestion • Pancreatic insufficiency • EFA deficiency • Fat digestion problems • Alkaline mineral insufficiency • Dental caries

Dr. Bieler's salivary pH acid challenge-
Identifying Imbalances in Secondary buffering systems

Normal patterns

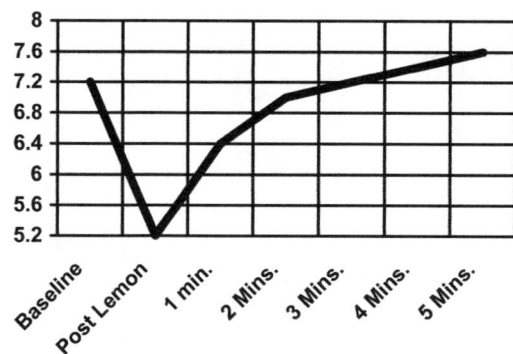

The initial salivary pH of 7.2 drops immediately after the acid challenge and takes a few minutes to climb up into the alkaline range. The slow climb up to 7.6 at 5 minutes indicates healthy mineral reserves

Baseline	Lemon	1	2	3	4	5
7.2	5.2	6.4	7.0	7.2	7.4	7.6

Alkaline Reaction

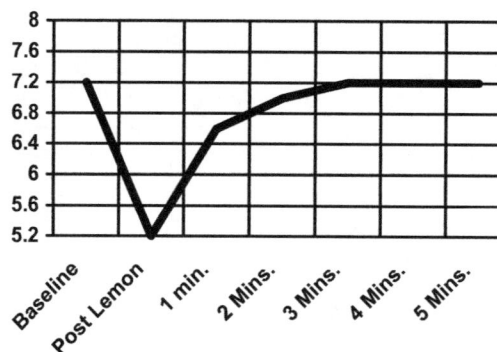

The alkaline reaction is a fairly normal reaction to a sudden increase of acid into the body but there are the beginnings of a tendency to drift towards mineral insufficiency. The Mineral reserves are intact but the buffering systems are not able to drive the pH as alkaline as the normal curve.

Baseline	Lemon	1	2	3	4	5
7.2	5.2	6.6	7.0	7.2	7.2	7.2

2. Mineral insufficiency

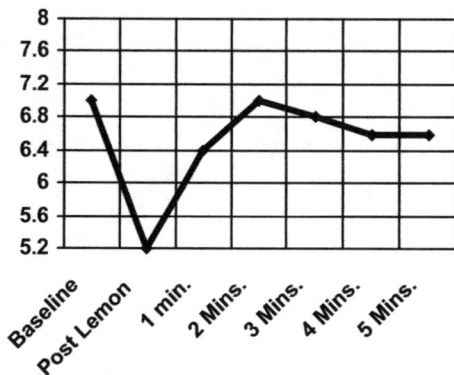

In the mineral insufficiency pattern the initial salivary pH of 7.2 drops immediately with the acid challenge and takes a few minutes to climb up to the alkaline range.

The slow climb up to a pH of 6.8 at 2 minutes starts to look like the normal curve, but it fails to completely alkalinize the saliva. This is an indication of mineral insufficiency. There are mineral reserves present but they are not replete enough to fully buffer the acidity.

The more the curve begins to drop the weaker the reserves are.

Baseline	Lemon	1	2	3	4	5
7.0	5.2	6.4	7.0	6.8	6.6	6.6

3. Hypersympathetic overload with mineral insufficiency

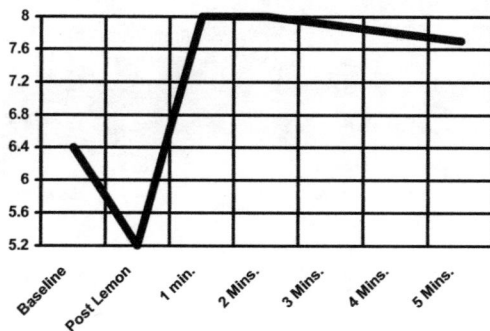

Starting point is acidic at 6.4. This pattern is already displaying signs of buffering problems before the test has started.

The alkaline spike after 1 minute indicates that ammonia is being used as a buffer. Ammonia, and not minerals, is being released. You may notice the ammonia response in the urine, which may have an ammonia smell.

This patient will complain of being wiped out and fatigued. They probably do not sleep well, are stressed and complain of feeling depleted. Any types of stress reduction techniques are essential for these people along with adrenal restoration. They often complain of not being able to relax. Notice also that the curve does not come down very quickly. The ammonia is quite a long term buffer.

Baseline	Lemon	1	2	3	4	5
6.4	5.2	8	8	7.9	7.8	7.7

4. Hypersympathetic overload with signs of mineral sufficiency

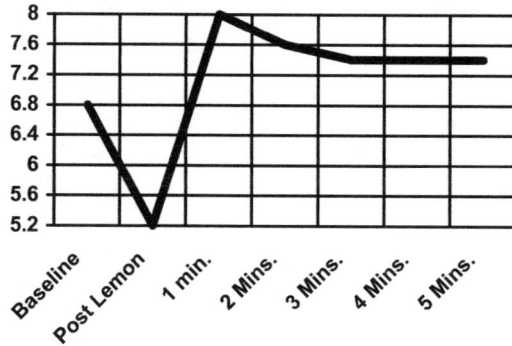

This curve looks similar to the curve above in the hyper sympathetic patient. There is still the ammonia spike but after 2 minutes there is signs of mineral reserve activity coming online because the pH is beginning to drop into the normal range.

Baseline	Lemon	1	2	3	4	5
6.8	5.2	8.0	7.6	7.4	7.4	7.4

5. Loss of alkaline reserves

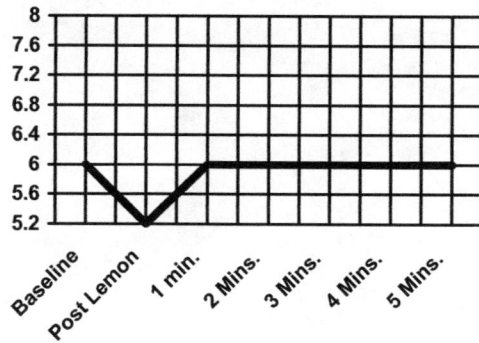

This pattern is an indication of a loss of buffering capacity, at least in the short term. There is probably cell rigidity and the kidneys are probably no longer reclaiming acidity. The first morning urine pH may be alkaline. Check the urine dipstick for any abnormalities and run a blood chemistry screen and CBC

Baseline	Lemon	1	2	3	4	5
6.0	5.2	6.0	6.0	6.0	6.0	6.0

Gastrointestinal Terrain

↑ Bowel Toxicity Test	↑ Sediment	Alkaline Gastro-test	↑ Urine Calcium
• Bowel toxemia • Dysbiosis • Hypochlorhydria • Maldigestion • Malabsorption • High protein intake	**Total**: • Poor assimilation • Pancreatic insufficiency • Leaky Gut Syndrome **Calcium phosphate:** • Carbohydrate, sugar and starch maldigestion **Uric acid:** • Protease deficiency • Hypochlorhydria • Protein maldigestion • Excess protein intake **Calcium oxalate:** • Fat maldigestion • Lipase deficiency • Poor fat emulsification • Calcium and magnesium deficiency ↓ **Total sediment** • Malabsorption	• Hypochlorhydria • Achlorhydria (>5.0) Use bicarbonate challenge to test acid reserves	• Excess calcium supplementation • Calcium mobilized from bone • High refined sugars in diet • Hyperparathyroidism ↓ **Urine calcium** • Low calcium in body • Excess protein intake • Malabsorption • Hypoparathyroidism

Hormonal Terrain

High Urine Chloride	Low Urine Chloride
• Adrenal hypofunctioning • Hypochlorhydria • Kidney stress • Alkaline mineral insufficiency • Oxidative stress	• Adrenal hyperfunction • Electrolyte stress/increased toxicity • Malabsorption syndrome • Diarrhea/excess vomiting

Oxidative Stress Terrain

Low Redox	+2 Oxidative stress	+3 Oxidative stress
<ul><li>Loss of high energy electron intermediates</li><li>Low electron potential</li><li>Susceptible to degenerative diseases</li><li>Premature tissue aging</li></ul>	<ul><li>Liver stress</li><li>Kidney stress</li><li>Pancreas stress</li><li>Blood sugar problems</li><li>Adrenal stress</li><li>Lymphatic congestion</li><li>Fatigue</li></ul>	<ul><li>Lymphatic stress</li><li>Xenotoxins</li><li>Greatly reduced ATP production</li><li>Maldigestion</li><li>Blood sugar dysregulation</li></ul>

The "Four Quadrants of Functional Diagnosis"
Diagnostic Education for the *Functional Age*

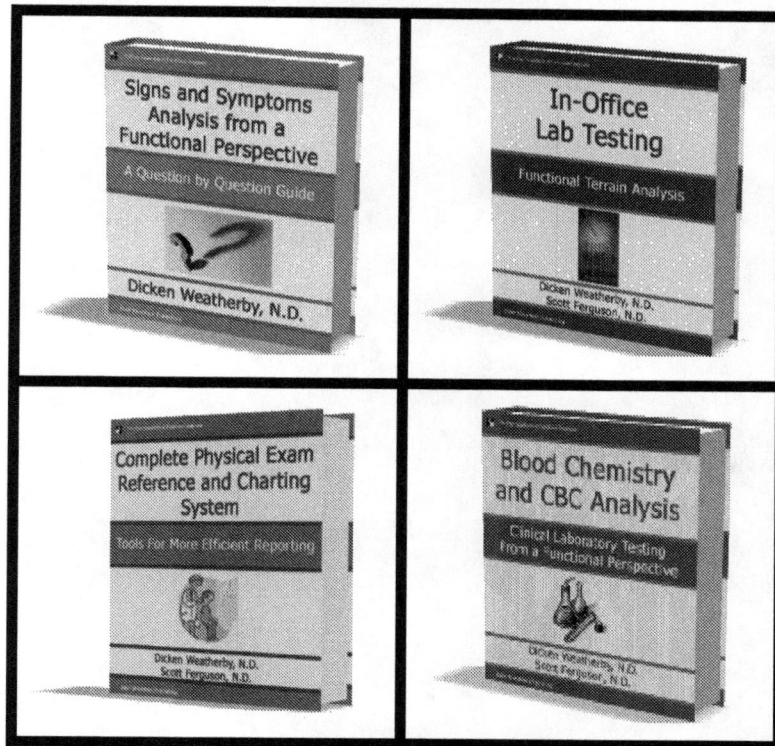

Most of us at some point or other have come to recognize that the diagnostic tests we learned in medical school taught us nothing about how to uncover our patients' functional problems. This is why I wrote my first book, *"Blood Chemistry and CBC Analysis- Clinical Laboratory Testing From a Functional Perspective"* with my colleague Dr. Scott Ferguson, to make the wealth of functional information you can get from a standard Chemistry Screen and CBC available to health care practitioners. This book and other products in my "Four Quadrants of Functional Diagnosis" series are designed to give you and your practice the same functional diagnostic education that thousands of practitioners have been using successfully in their practices.

The *Four Quadrants of Functional Diagnosis* will help you:
- Get excellent patient results
- Dramatically improve your clinical outcomes
- Get more referrals
- Cut the amount of time you spend analyzing your patient cases
- Set up a system of functional tests that will be the envy of all your colleagues

In preparing for the Functional Age, the rules on how to manage the diagnostic information in your practice have changed. You can no longer blindly use the same tests every one else is using and hope to get different results. The Functional Age will require that you have more information to be able to properly find the cause of your patients' problems. *Signs and Symptoms Analysis from A Functional Perspective, Boost Clinic Income With an In-Office Lab System,* and *The Functional Blood Chemistry Analysis System* were developed for practitioners just like you who recognize the need for a new paradigm in diagnostic information. Practitioners who realize that the Pathological Age is over and the Functional Age has begun.

Dr. Dicken Weatherby, Naturopathic Physician

Functional Blood Chemistry Analysis

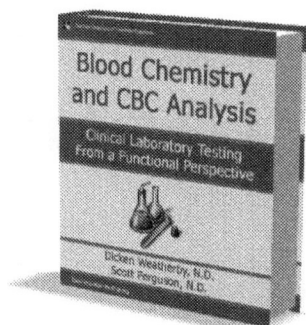

Blood Chemistry and CBC Analysis- Clinical Laboratory Testing from a Functional Perspective

This book presents a diagnostic system of blood chemistry and CBC analysis that focuses on physiological function as a marker of health. By looking for optimum function we increase our ability to detect dysfunction long before disease manifests. Conventional lab testing becomes a truly preventative and prognostic tool. A must for any practitioners who wants to get more from the tests they are already running.

Printed Book $65.00 (in the U.S.A.) ISBN: 0-9761367-1-6

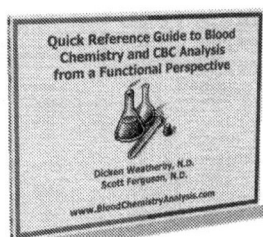

Quick Reference Guide to Blood Chemistry Analysis From a Functional Perspective

This guide is the perfect companion to our Blood Chemistry and CBC Analysis Book. It is a complete reference for interpreting, analyzing, and finding the underlying cause of your patients' functional complaints. You will find yourself referring to this guide over and over again.

Printed Book $35.00 (in the U.S.A.) ISBN: 0-9761367-8-3

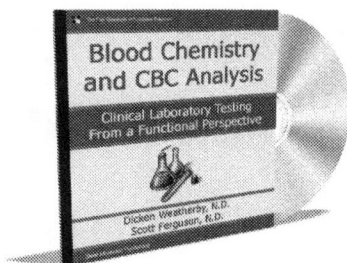

Functional Blood Chemistry Analysis Seminar on Audio

Any practitioners of the healing arts will gain a tremendous benefit from listening to this complete one day seminar on audio CD. Dr. Weatherby guides the listener through his method of analyzing blood chemistry and CBC tests. Topics include using standard blood tests to analyze the following: GI dysfunction, minerals and vitamin insufficiencies, blood sugar dysregulation, cardiovascular problems, thyroid issues, and adrenal dysfunction..

6 hours of audio $147.00 (in the U.S.A.) ISBN: 0-9726469-4-9

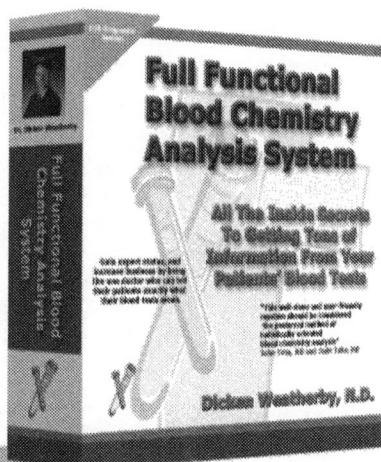

The Full Functional Blood Chemistry Analysis System is a complete road map to success that shows you exactly how to approach each blood chemistry analysis step by step. This system includes the printed reference book, the Quick Reference Guide, and the Audio Recordings, a system for getting the most out of your blood chemistry tests.

A functional diagnosis of your patients' blood test results is one of the most effective diagnostic tools to get to the bottom of the myriad of health complaints your patients present with. Gain expert status, and increase business by being the one doctor who can tell patients exactly what their blood tests mean.

Full Blood Chemistry System $197.00 (in the U.S.A.) ISBN: 0-9761367-3-2

In-Office Lab Testing
Boost Your Clinic Income!

I want you to be successful in your practice and to have the same tools that I use to increase clinical efficacy and clinic income, which is why I created my *Boost Clinic Income With an In-Office Lab System.* The tests I present in this system will help you get a wealth of functional data from your patients and the income you make on these tests stays in your practice. At the heart of this system is my Functional Urinalysis program.

Functional Urinalysis allows you to run a series of simple urine tests that get to the heart of the disturbances in your patients' inner "terrain". These tests have been used for many years but until now the interpretive information available to health care practitioners has been poor. I have put together the most comprehensive system for understanding and interpreting the Functional Urinalysis. Watch the instructional DVD, listen to the 2 audio CDs packed with time saving tips and interpretive tools, refer to the in-depth reference manual, and start paying for your office overhead with Functional Urinalysis!

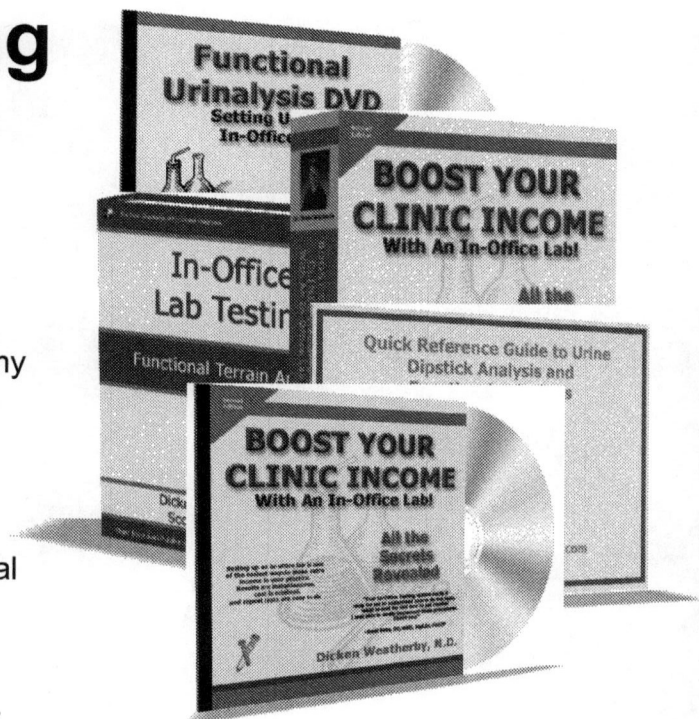

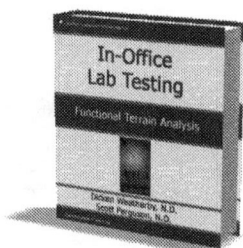

Reference Manual
$85.00 (in the U.S.A)
ISBN: 0-9761367-4-0

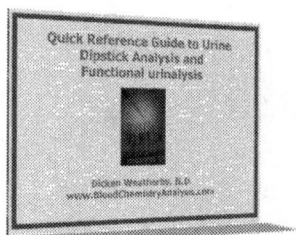

Urine Dipstick Guide
$35.00 (in the U.S.A)
ISBN: 0-9761367-9-1

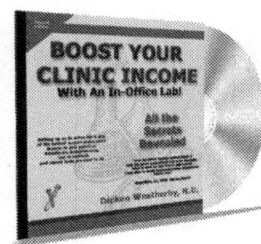

Functional Urinalysis
Audio Program
$85.00 (in the U.S.A)

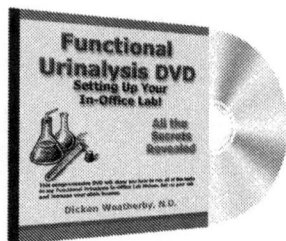

Functional Urinalysis DVD
$85.00 (in the U.S.A)

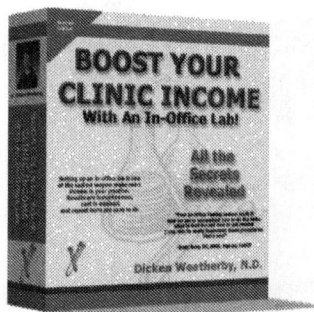

Get the complete **"Boost Clinic Income With an In-Office Lab"** system to rapidly increase your clinic income with Functional Urinalysis and other in-office labs. Save $43.00 by getting all the above tools bundled together.
$247.00 (in the U.S.A)
ISBN: 09726469-1-4

Other Functional Diagnostic Tools

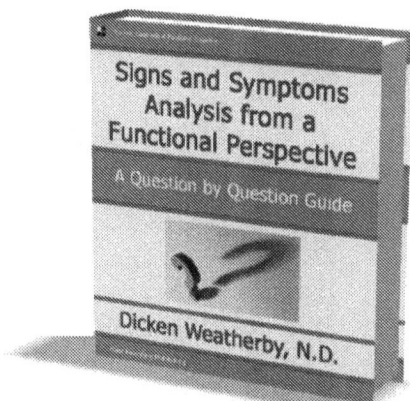

Signs and Symptoms Analysis From a Functional Perspective

This book takes a critical look at the myriad of signs and symptoms a patient presents with. Using a comprehensive signs and symptoms questionnaire you can look at the symptom burden in specific systems of the body, address some of the more obscure symptoms, and track changes over time. Organized by body systems, this book provides the nutritional and functional explanations behind the 322 questions on Dr. Weatherby's 4-page questionnaire.

Printed Book $65.00 (in the U.S.A.) ISBN: 0-9761367-2-4

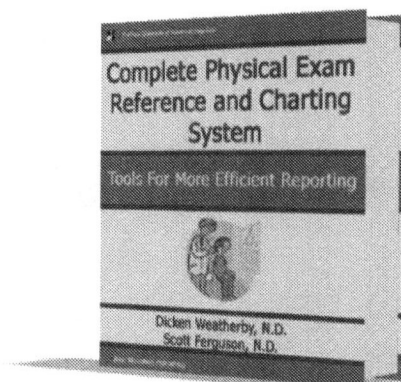

Complete PE Reference and Charting System

Drs. Weatherby and Ferguson have put together report forms for all the major physical examinations commonly performed in your office (i.e. cardiovascular, lung, abdominal, neurological examinations). These report forms provide an easy method of charting and filing your physical examination results.

The accompanying reference cards fit neatly into your white coat and provide a detailed explanation of all the tests on each report form and are an excellent "exam-side" reference to refresh your memory on all the different tests that make up each examination.

Printed Reference Cards and CD $65.00 (in the U.S.A.)

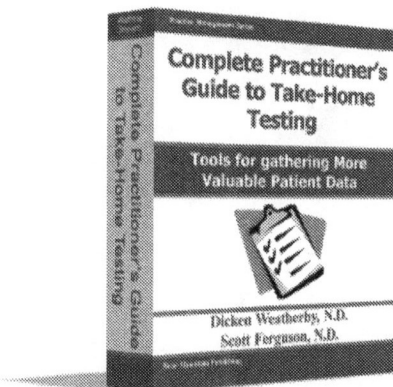

Complete Practitioner's Guide to Take-Home Testing

Drs. Weatherby and Ferguson have put together a series of 17 take-home tests that you can give to your patients to perform in between their office visits. These tests will allow you to assess for digestion, elimination, zinc status, pH regulation, hypothyroid conditions, iodine insufficiency, blood type, and food and other sensitivities and intolerances. Patient "homework" is an important method of gathering patient data and encouraging compliance.

Printed Book $45.00 (in the U.S.A.) ISBN: 0-9761367-7-5

Quick Order Form

Fax Orders: 541-488-0323. Send this form.

Telephone orders: Call 541-482-3779

Email orders: orders@bBloodChemistryAnalysis.com

Secure online orders: http://www.BloodChemistryAnalysis.com/diagnosisshop.html

Postal orders: Weatherby & Associates, LLC, 2693 Takelma Way, Ashland, OR 97520, USA. Telephone: 541-482-3779

Please send the following books, CDs or reports. I understand that I may return any of them for a full refund – for any reason, no questions asked.

_____
_____
_____

Please send more FREE information on:

☐ Other books ☐ Live Seminars or Teleseminars ☐ Speaking ☐ Consulting

Name:_____

Address:_____

City:_____ State: _____ Zip:_____

Phone:_____ E-mail:_____

Shipping by air
US: $4.00 for first book and $2.00 for each additional product.
International: $9.00 for first book; $5.00 for each additional product (estimate)

Payment: ☐ Cheque   ☐ Credit Card
☐ Visa   ☐ Mastercard   ☐ AMEX   ☐ Discover

Personal check (payable to Weatherby & Associates, LLC):

Card number:_____

Name on card:_____ Exp. Date:_____

http://www.BloodChemistryAnalysis.com